Pure Soap Making:

Beginners Guide On How To Create Your Own Natural Soap

+ 31 Amazing Homemade Soap Recipes

Table of content:

Introduction

Research suggests that soap was being used as long ago as 2800 B.C. The ancient Babylonians are thought to have made soap from ashes and fat, although it is unknown as to the extent that soap was used by the general population.

There is also evidence to suggest that the Ancient Egyptians, from approximately 1500 B.C. used a soap product created by mixing fatty animal oils with salt; in effect to create a soap which would exfoliate as well! Even the Romans are known to have made a form of soap from urine!

Soap is, in effect a vital part of human history, whether washing the blood from your hands in ancient times or destroying microscopic germs; it has always been used. Of course, the more modern versions of soap have been created to leave a pleasant aroma as well as effective and gently washing the skin.

As with most products, soap was originally something that only the richest people could afford; there were very few people capable or licensed to make soap, and they guarded their skills carefully. Mainly used animal oil and parts of plants to create distinctive soaps. This ensured an elite class of customer. However, at the end of the 18th century, a Frenchman discovered a way of chemical making soap; this was the first time soap could be made on a much larger scale. This was the catalyst which drove the price of soap down and made it affordable to a much wider range of people.

This discovery was followed in the early part of the 19th century that soap could be made from glycerin, fats, and acid. This made it even cheaper to create soap and is considered to be the foundations of modern soap making; there have been no significant advancements in the science of soap making since.

The techniques and principles which were first used approximately two hundred years ago are still in use today!

Of course, modern technology has changed the understanding of soap, the ingredients are better understood and broken down which has enabled the creation of different types of soap for different situations. Laundry soap is one example of a product which is subtly different to hand soap or even bathing soaps; each has its role to fulfill. It was only in the 1970's that liquid soap became possible; it has become exceptionally popular since and helps to promote hand washing as well as minimize soap wastage.

The modern world has a dazzling array if soaps, depending upon your needs, how you wish to smell and even what type of skin you have. These constant changes, improvements, and marketing ploys help to keep soap fresh in everyone's mind; a standard bar of soap may be less popular, but the concept and use of soaps have never been so popular. There remains a thriving market for commercially created soaps; there is also a place for those who wish to create their own, homemade soap; a process which I surprisingly easy!

This book will guide you through the best method to make soap and the tools and equipment you will need to complete this task at home. It will also provide you with a selection of 31 recipes to help you practice and create your soap; you should then be able to discover and make hundreds of other types of soap!

Chapter 1 – The Need For Soap and How to Make It

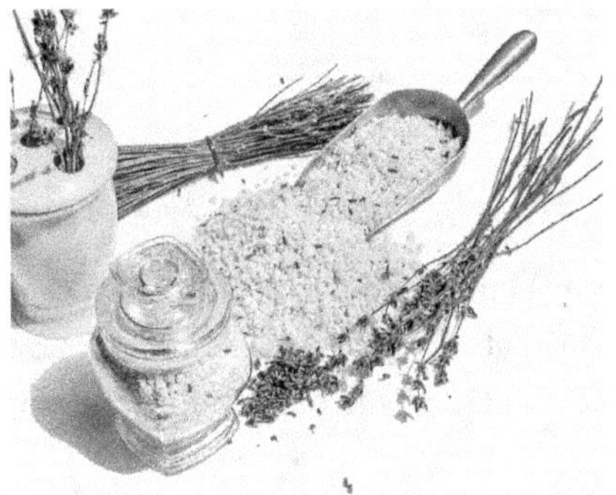

In the modern world, everyone is aware of the need for soap and its role in helping us to stay clean and healthy, although many people are unaware of how soap works and how regularly it should be used. In fact, there have been many studies on the effects of soap. There are even those who believe that soap is not necessary; the body can clean itself. There are two main uses of soap:

Odor Removal

In general, research agrees that young children, male or female do not have any odor creating regions. It is, therefore, not necessary for children to use soap to remove unpleasant body odors, although soap can still be used to aid them in smelling nice. However, adults, particularly men, do have odor producing regions. Research suggests that it is essential to soap these regions every two days unless you partake in very physical work; in which case every day is essential. Water by itself can significantly reduce the presence if body odor, but will not eliminate it.

Deodorant will always be needed to assist with reducing and containing odors, the regularity of application will be directly related to the physical duties undertaken. Washing in water will help to reduce body odor but it is more effective when mixed with soap.

Cleanliness

Soap has always been acknowledged as a way to remove dirt and germs from your hands; this is via a process of friction and agitation; in fact, modern soaps have small particles added to them to aid with dirt removal and the removal of excess skin.

The abrasive nature of these products will help to leave your skin fresh and glowing and will often help to keep skin conditions at bay. This is because many soap products are becoming more technologically advanced and can offer deep-pore washes.

It is the amount of science behind the soap that often worries people regarding what they are putting on their face or body. This is one of the main reasons people start to make their soap; knowing which ingredients have been placed into a bar means you know what you are putting on your body.

The basic process of making any soap is surprisingly simple, in fact, the most important question you will need to ask yourself is whether you wish to handle Lye yourself or not. Lye is a natural product, also known as Sodium Hydroxide. It is an alkali and can be dangerous; it is capable of making a hole in your fabrics and can burn your skin. However, as long as you handle it with care there will be no issue using it; it is worth noting that you should always use the crystal version of Lye when making salt and it must always be added to the water, not the water to it.

This lye, added in the right quantities to plain water can then be mixed with a variety of different oil. The mixture bonds together to create soap; the main difference between recipes is the additional flavorings and the type of oil used. Every oil has its own specific relationship to lye and must be used in the right quantities.

If the thought of handling lye is too daunting for you at first, then you can purchase a melt and pour soap which is ready to use. As its name suggests, you simply melt it, add your own flavors and pour it into the molds.

Chapter 2 – Cold Processed Soaps

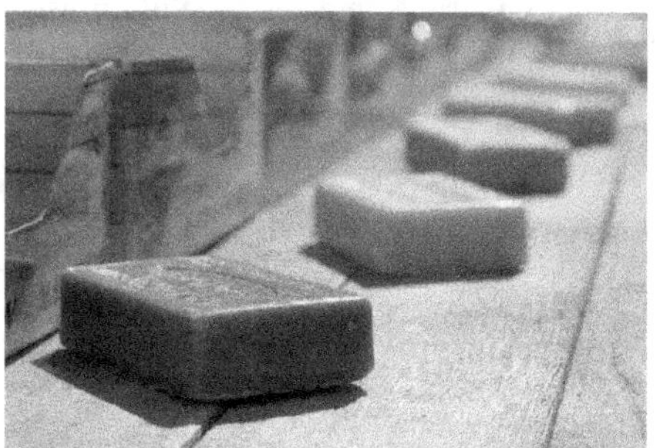

What you will soon discover is that it is entirely possible for you to create your soap recipes from scratch. All you need is a few simple guidelines, and you can formulate your blends using your favorite oils and additives. In this section, we have provided for you three basic soap formulas that you can build off of and modify if you choose to once you feel comfortable. You can create almost any soap you desire from these fundamental methods. Following the basic recipes, you will find a selection of solvents that are crafted for different uses and preferences. Each one has in some way been built off of one of the basic recipes. You can craft amazing soaps with one of these recipes, or use them as inspiration to create your special formula bars.

Basic Vegetable Soap

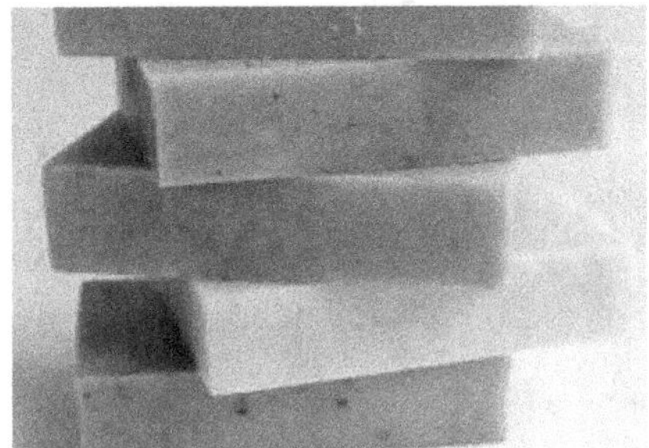

This base recipe is designed to give you everything you want in a bar soap. The latter is rich, and it is mild and conditioning. A perfect bar for every skin type including very sensitive skin. Yields 15-20 five-ounce bars of soap.

Ingredients:

- 250g coconut oil
- 500g palm oil
- 500g olive oil
- 380g distilled water
- 186.25g lye

Directions:

1. Follow the instructions for making cold processed soaps.
2. Insulate for twenty-four hours and check every day for hardness. When the soap is firm, remove from the molds and allow curing for at least two weeks before using.

No Palm Vegetable Soap

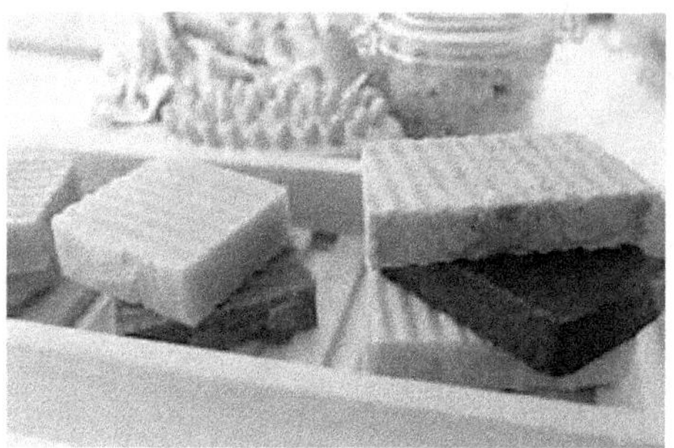

This is a great long-lasting, all-purpose soap for people who prefer to not use palm oil for environmental concerns. It can be used for skin care as well as household cleaning purposes. Yields 15-20 five-ounce bars of soap.

Ingredients:

- 250g coconut oil
- 500g olive oil
- 600g vegetable shortening
- 400g distilled water
- 197g lye

Directions:

1. Follow the instructions for making cold processed soaps.
2. Insulate for twenty-four hours and check every day for hardness. When the soap is firm, remove from the molds and allow to cure for at least two weeks before using. As you are starting out, it is a good idea to include

Basic Animal Fat Soap

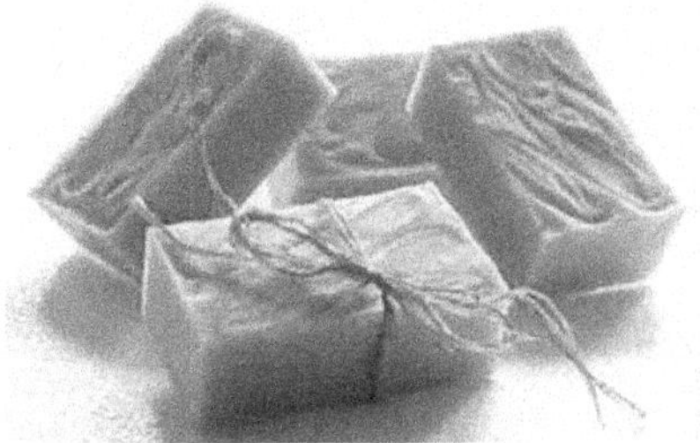

This is the longest lasting, firmest, and mildest bar among the basic formulas. People with sensitive skin will find animal fat soaps to be the least irritating of soap formulas. This particular bar produces a mild, milky, and conditioning lather that can be used everywhere from the shower to the kitchen and even in the laundry room. Yields 15-20 five-ounce bars of soap.

Ingredients:

- 500g beef tallow
- 700g lard
- 350g distilled water
- 168g lye

Directions:

1. Follow the instructions for making cold processed soaps.
2. Insulate for twenty-four hours and check every day for hardness. When the soap is firm, remove from the molds and allow to cure for at least two weeks before using.

Kitchen and Bath Hand Soap

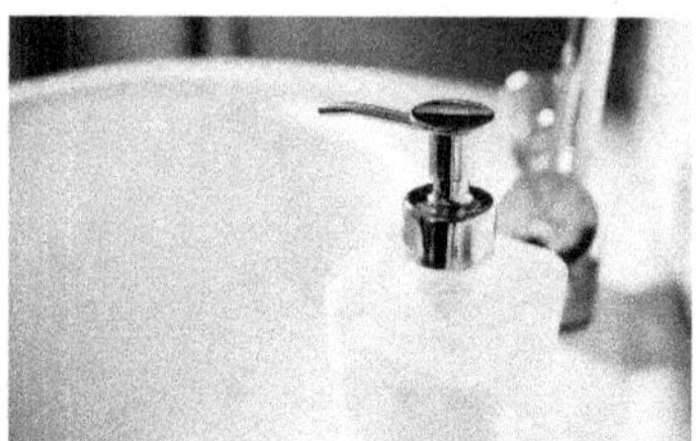

This big lathering soap contains beeswax and olive oil to keep skin soft and smooth while the brewed coffee added works as an odor eliminator that is perfect for removing string food smells from your hands. Yields 15-20 five-ounce bars of soap.

Ingredients:

* 250g coconut oil
* 500g palm oil
* 600g olive oil
* 150g castor oil
* 50g beeswax
* 440g cold brewed coffee made with distilled water
* 219g lye

Directions:

1. Follow the instructions for making cold processed soaps.
2. Add the beeswax when the soap traces.
3. Insulate for twenty-four hours and check every day for hardness. When the soap is firm, remove from the molds and allow to cure for at least two weeks before using.

Soothing Face Soap

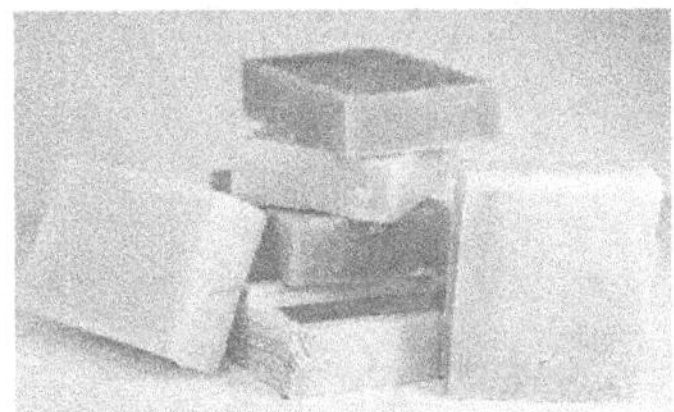

With tallow as a base, this soap is a gentle soap to use on the delicate facial skin. Shea butter, oatmeal, and lavender add additional soothing and softening properties to this mildly scented and therapeutic bar. Yields 15-20 five-ounce bars of soap.

Ingredients:

- 300g beef tallow
- 350g olive oil
- 70g castor oil
- 100g shea butter
- 50g ground oatmeal
- 25g dried lavender, finely ground
- 225g distilled water
- 111g lye

Directions:

1. Follow the instructions for making cold processed soaps.
2. Add the dried lavender and oatmeal when the soap traces.
3. Insulate for twenty-four hours and check every day for hardness. When the soap is firm, remove from the molds and allow to cure for at least two weeks before using.

All-Purpose Shower and Bath Bar

This soap produces a nice strong, thick lather while the goat's milk and shea butter are extra moisturizing. This bar is perfect for use on the entire body including the face, hair, and even as an in-shower shave bar. The Earl Grey tea infused offers a delicate scent and light color to the bar. Yields 15-20 five-ounce bars of soap.

Ingredients:

- 300g coconut oil
- 300g palm oil
- 550g olive oil
- 150g castor oil
- 100g shea butter
- 25g dried lavender, finely ground
- 2 ounces lavender essential oil
- 6 ounces goat's milk
- 1-ounce earl grey tea
- 412g distilled water
- 206g lye

Directions:

1. Steep the Earl Grey tea in 22.0g of the included distilled water.
2. The goat's milk should be chilled to a slush consistency.
3. Follow the instructions for making cold processed soaps.
4. Add the goat's milk to the oils once the oils reach 110°F/43°C.
5. The Earl Grey tea, ground lavender, and lavender essential oil are added at trace.
6. Insulate for twenty-four hours and check every day for hardness. When the soap is firm, remove from the molds and allow to cure for at least two weeks before using.

Basic Face and Shave Bar

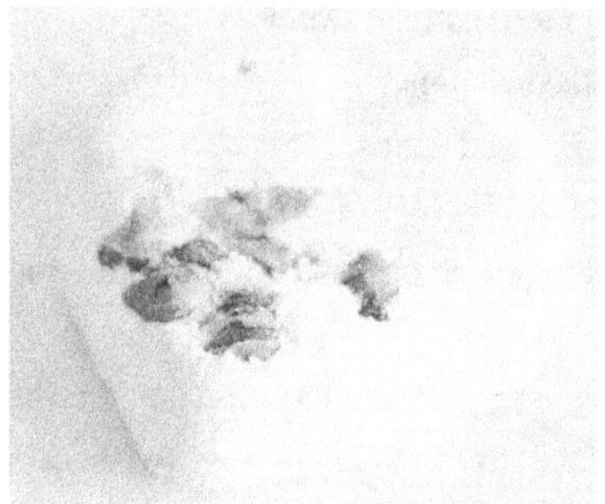

This face and shave bar produces a good lather while the castor oil adds extra glycerin to the soap. This combined with the glide provided by the clay and the repairing and moisturizing properties of the beeswax and shea butter makes a rich, moisturizing soap that will leave your face and body soothed, even after a shave. Yields 15-20 five-ounce bars of soap.

Ingredients:

- 200g coconut oil
- 300g vegetable shortening
- 400g olive oil
- 150g castor oil
- 40g bentonite clay (added at trace)
- 25g beeswax
- 100g shea butter
- 336g distilled water
- 167g lye

Directions:

1. Follow the instructions for making cold processed soaps.
2. Insulate for twenty-four hours and check every day for hardness. When the soap is firm, remove from the molds and allow to cure for at least two weeks before using.

Masculine Face and Shave Bar

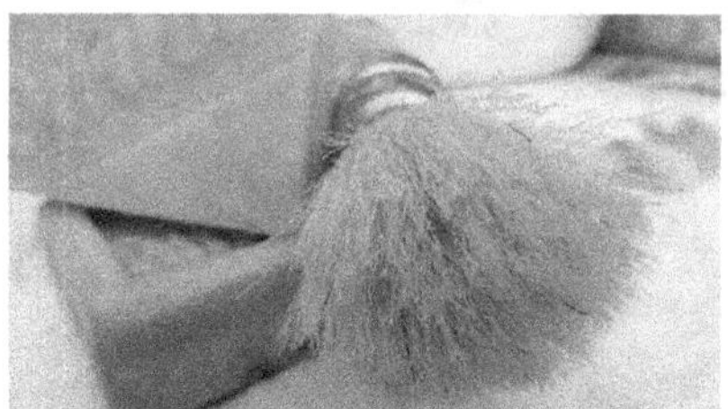

A shave bar created specifically for men, the coconut oil, castor oil and the IPA produces a big thick lather. The hemp oil provides a light, nutty oil but also offers a moisturizing and repairing component that is rich in vitamins and healing to the skin. The clay adds a glide that allows your shaver to slide smoothly over the skin. The hops are softening to facial hair and also have antibacterial properties, so it acts preventatively in healing any tiny nicks or abrasions that may occur. Yields 15-20 five-ounce bars of soap.

Ingredients:

- 300g beef tallow
- 300g olive oil
- 150g coconut oil
- 150g castor oil
- 200g hemp oil
- 100g shea butter
- 25g liquid vitamin e
- 50g bentonite clay
- 25g fresh ground hops
- 342g IPA (beer)
- 170g lye

Directions:

In this formula, the beer replaces the water. For best results, a day or two before making the soap, pour the beer into a large mason jar. A couple of times a day, shake the jar, and once the foam settles, open it slowly and remove the lid for thirty minutes to an hour. It will eliminate the carbonation in the beer. Too much carbonation can be a hazard during the soap making process, so it is best to remove it as much as possible. Some soap makers prefer to cook off the alcohol in the beer, which will also lessen the carbonation, however, this is not necessary as long as you are using a beer that is of typical alcohol content.

1. Follow the instructions for making cold processed soaps.
2. Add the vitamin E, bentonite clay and hops trace.
3. Insulate for twenty-four hours and check every day for hardness. When the soap is firm, remove from the molds and allow to cure for at least two weeks before using.

Country Pantry Soap

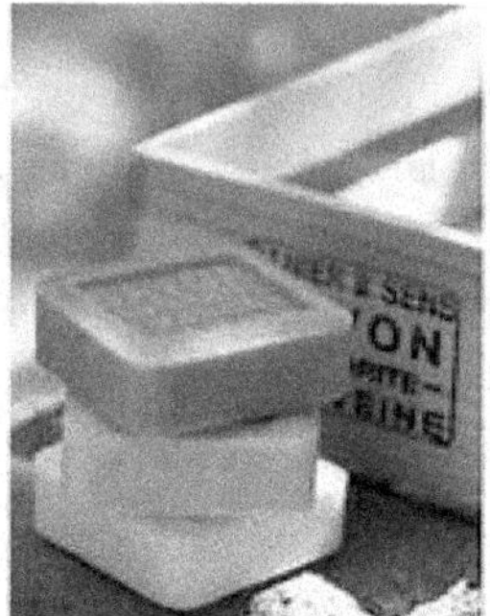

A simple, basic soap made from most oils that you would find in any small grocery store or country pantry. Nothing fancy here and no outside suppliers needed. These oils produce a nice, conditioning bar of soap. Yields 15-20 five-ounce bars of soap.

Ingredients:

- 850g lard
- 250g corn oil
- 500g olive oil
- 250g canola oil
- 506g distilled water
- 252g lye

Directions:

1. Follow the instructions for making cold processed soaps.
2. Insulate for twenty-four hours and check every day for hardness. When the soap is firm, remove from the molds and allow to cure for at least two weeks before using.

City Pantry Soap

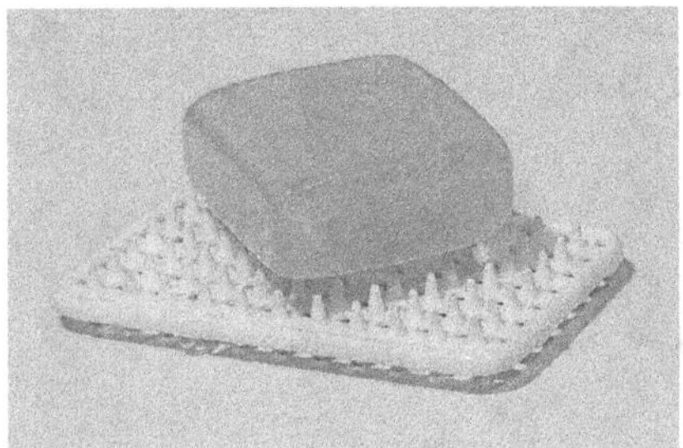

Much like the Country Pantry Soap, the City Pantry Soap shows you how you can make a perfect, all-purpose bar of soap from ingredients that are inexpensive and easy to find with a single trip to your supermarket. Yields 15-20 five-ounce bars of soap.

Ingredients:

- 250g coconut oil
- 300g olive oil
- 250g soya bean oil
- 400g vegetable shortening
- 356g distilled water
- 177g lye

Directions:

1. Follow the instructions for making cold processed soaps.
2. Insulate for twenty-four hours and check every day for hardness. When the solvent is firm, remove from the molds and allow to cure for at least two weeks before using.

Winter Facial Bar

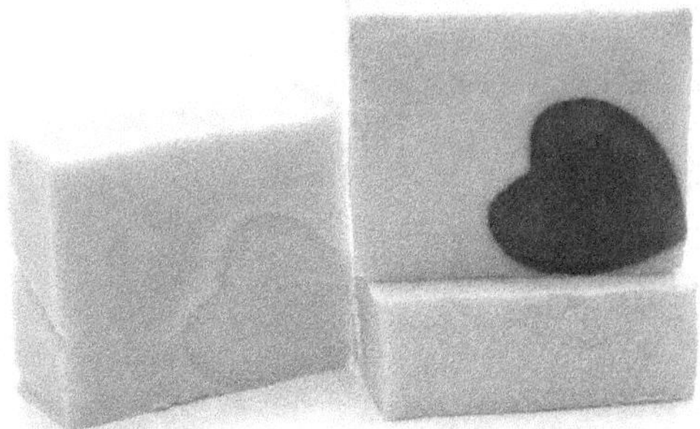

This method is a take on the Swedish Egg White Soap that is famed for keeping women's skin soft and smooth during the harsh winter environment. Vitamin E adds antioxidants to the soap to further protect delicate facial skin. The rose water and rose oil are both soothing and refreshing. Yields 15-20 five-ounce bars of soap.

Ingredients:

- 300g palm oil
- 200g coconut oil
- 600g olive oil
- 3 egg whites
- 50g vitamin e oil
- 1 ounce rose essential oil or rose absolute
- 325g rose water
- 161.8g lye

Directions:

1. Follow the instructions for making cold processed soaps.

2. Rose water takes the place of regular distilled water in this recipe.

3.   Temper the egg whites with a little warm olive oil so that they do not scramble when added at trace.

4.   It is best to not make this soap at a temperature exceeding 120°F/49°C. It will also help keep the integrity of the egg whites.

5. Add the egg whites, vitamin E and rose essential oil at trace.

6.   Insulate for twenty-four hours and check every day for hardness. When the soap is firm, remove from the molds and allow to cure for at least two weeks before using.

Summer Lime Bar

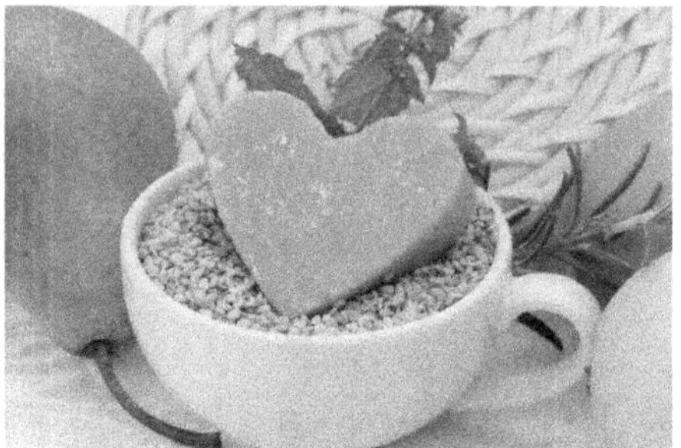

This is a basic vegetable bar recipe with added moisturizers to help repair parched, damaged summer skin. The avocado oil, cocoa butter, and vitamin E help to heal and protect while the lime zest and essential oils provide a soothing and refreshing scent. Yields 15-20 five-ounce bars.

Ingredients:

- 250g coconut oil
- 300g palm oil
- 500g olive oil
- 150g avocado oil
- 100g cocoa butter
- 30g vitamin E
- 2 tablespoons lime zest
- 2 tablespoons dried lavender, ground
- 1-ounce sandalwood essential oil
- 1-ounce cypress essential oil
- 390g distilled water
- 191.5g lye

Directions:

1. Follow the instructions for making cold processed soaps.
2. Add the vitamin E with the main oils.
3. Add the lime zest, dried lavender, and essential oils at trace.
4. Insulate for twenty-four hours and check every day for hardness. When the soap is firm, remove from the molds and allow to cure for at least two weeks before using.

Herbal Shampoo Bar

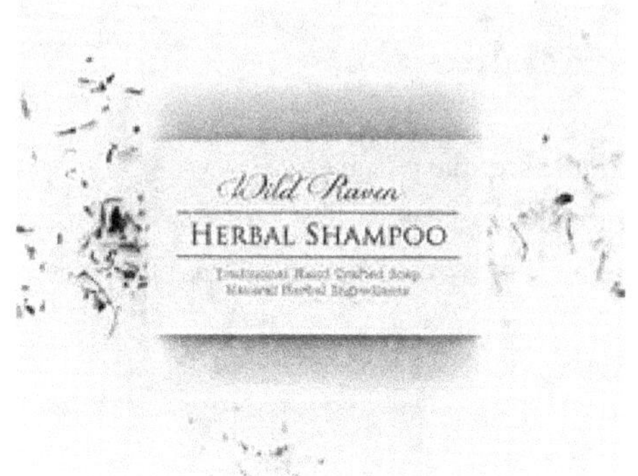

There is another example of how to use one of the basic formulas to create a specialized soap to suit your needs. The hemp and jojoba oils help to condition the hair. Hops are added for their famed hair beautifying qualities and rosemary helps to soothe an irritated scalp and prevents dry scalp skin. Yields 15-20 five-ounce bars.

Ingredients:

- 250g coconut oil
- 300g palm oil
- 500g olive oil
- 100g hemp seed oil
- 75g jojoba oil
- 1-ounce lavender essential oils
- 1-ounce rosemary essential oil
- 2 tablespoons ground hops
- 360g distilled water
- 176g lye

Directions:

1.   Place the ground hops in a tea ball or infuser and make a tea infusion with the hops and distilled water. Let the hops steep for twenty-four hours. Remove the ground hops from the tea bag and reserve.
2.   Follow the instructions for making cold processed soaps.
3.   Add the reserved ground hops, lavender essential oil, and rosemary essential oil at trace.
4.   Insulate for twenty-four hours and check every day for hardness. When the soap is firm, remove from the molds and allow to cure for at least two weeks before using.

Invigorating Foot Soap

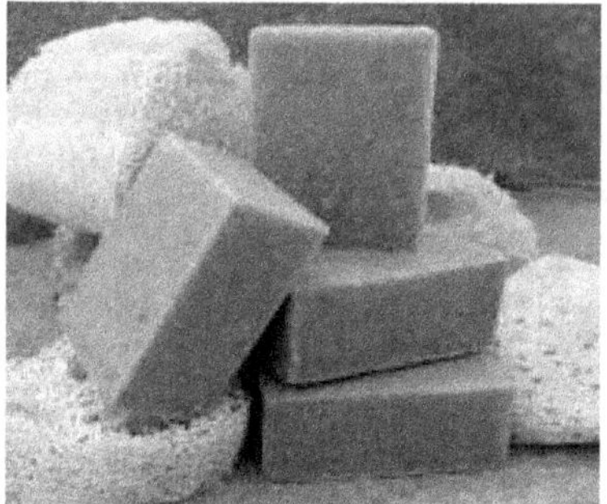

This citrusy soap is mild with a white lather to help soothe the skin. The coffee added provides a gentle exfoliant. This bar will leave your feet soft, smooth and refreshed. Yields 15-20 five-ounce bars of soap.

Ingredients:

- 300g beef tallow
- 150g shea butter
- 50g beeswax
- 400g olive oil
- 100g avocado oil
- 2 tablespoons coarse ground coffee
- 1 teaspoon orange zest
- 1 teaspoon lemon zest
- 1 teaspoon lime zest
- 315g distilled water
- 154.25g lye

Directions:

1. Follow the instructions for making cold processed soaps.
2. Add the ground coffee, orange zest, lemon zest, and lime zest at trace.
3. Insulate for twenty-four hours and check every day for hardness. When the soap is firm, remove from the molds and allow to cure for at least two weeks before using.

Her Shave Soap

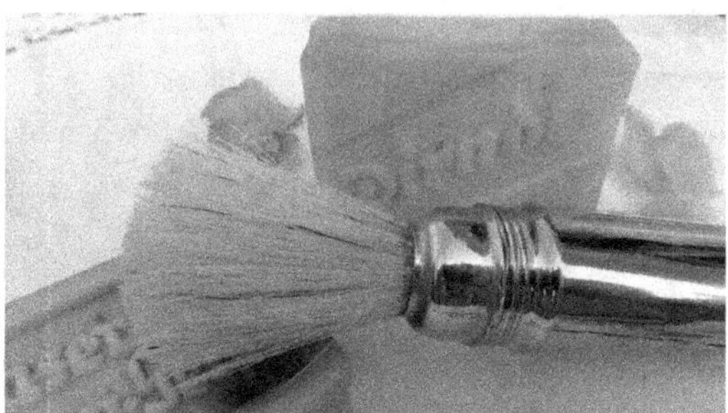

A very mild shave soap that will produce fine, thick and moisturizing lather. The glycerin and honey protect the skin and the clay provides a nice glide for a razor. This soap is mild and conditioning enough to use for daily shaving purposes. Yields 15-20 five-ounce bars of soap.

Ingredients:

- 400g beef tallow
- 400g olive oil
- 75g jojoba oil
- 100g shea butter
- 100g wheat germ oil
- 50g glycerin
- 30g bentonite clay
- 30g honey
- 1-ounce chamomile essential oil
- 1-ounce lavender essential oil
- 330g distilled water
- 163.25g lye

Directions:

1. Follow the instructions for making cold processed soaps.

2. Add the glycerin, bentonite clay, honey, chamomile essential oil, and lavender essential oil at trace.

3. Insulate for twenty-four hours and check every day for hardness. When the soap is firm, remove from the molds and allow to cure for at least two weeks before using.

Old-Fashioned Pine Tar Soap

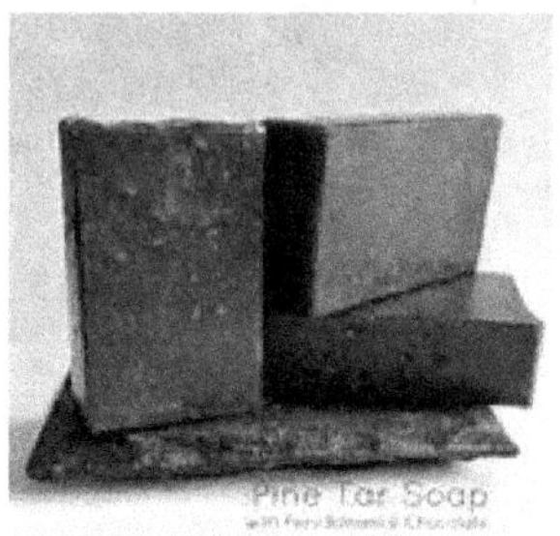

This nostalgic DIY soap is the answer to dry, itchy skin, eczema, dandruff, and psoriasis.

Ingredients:

- 13.5 oz. lard
- 13.5 oz. olive oil
- 8.2 oz. palm kernel oil
- 5.8 oz. sunflower oil
- 7.2 oz. pine tar
- 5.9 oz. lye
- 15.8 oz. water
- 2 oz. lavender, tea tree, eucalyptus, and Siberian fir essential oil blend
- 1 tbsp. sugar added to the water for the lye solution, before you add the lye

Directions:

Follow the Cold Process Soap Making method.

Peppermint and Rosemary Soap

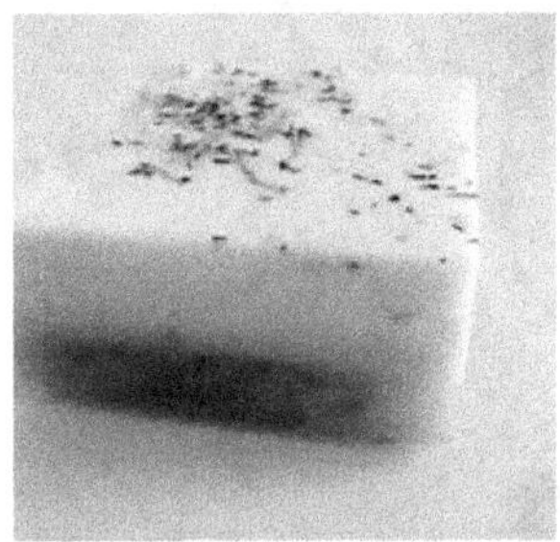

Ingredients:

- 15 oz. olive oil
- 13 oz. coconut oil
- 2.6 oz. castor oil
- 16 oz. distilled water
- 6.2 oz. lye
- 0.8 oz. peppermint essential oil
- 0.8 rosemary essential oil
- 0.4 oz. sage essential oil
- ¼ oz. spirulina
- 1 oz. dried peppermint leaves

Directions:

Follow the Cold Process Soap Making method.

Aloe Vera Soap

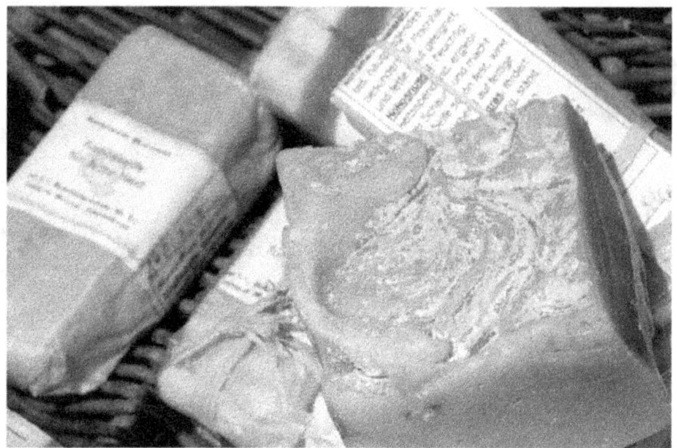

Ingredients:

- 15 oz. refined coconut oil
- 13.5 oz. extra virgin olive oil
- 10.5 oz. lard
- 2.5 oz. organic shea butter
- 10 oz. aloe vera gel and water puree
- 6.5 oz. lye
- 10 oz. purified water

Directions:

Use the Cold Process Soap Making method.

Winter Rose Soap

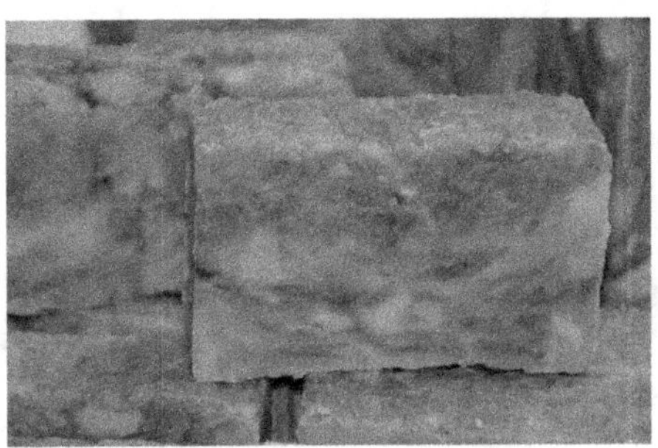

Ingredients:

- 28 oz. refined coconut oil
- 42 oz. extra virgin olive oil
- 12 oz. sunflower oil
- 11.73 oz. Lye
- 26 oz. strained rose petal infusion (create a tea)
- At trace, stir in 1 tablespoon each of rosehip seed oil, jojoba oil and melted shea butter. (optional, makes a higher superfatted bar)
- Also at trace, add a few teaspoons geranium essential oil.

Directions:

Use the Cold Process Soap Making method for this recipe.

Chapter 3 – Melt and Pour Soaps

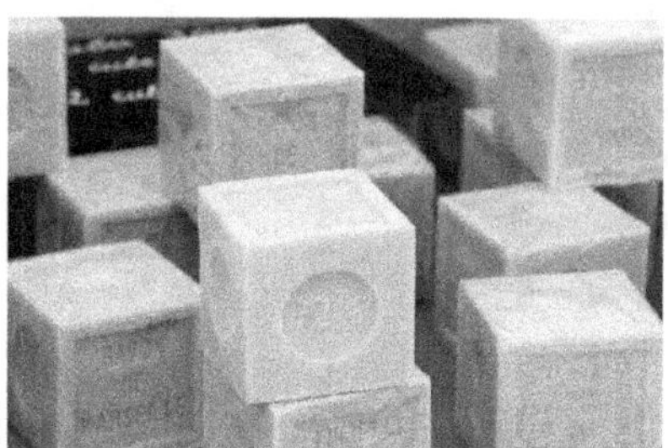

Here you will find some incredibly simple ideas for personalizing melt and pour glycerin soap bases. You will find that these recipes are given in volume measurements rather than the weight measurements used in making cold processed soaps. This is because with melt and pours soap, and you do not depend on a chemical reaction to occur for the soap to form. Therefore, the units of measurement do not need to be as precise. While these recipes inspire you, the reality is that the sky is the limit with melt and pour soaps. Let your imagination run wild.

*As a side note, we have not included any rebatch or hand-milled recipes in this book, as those depend significantly upon what type of soap you are using to rebatch as well as the already existing ingredients. You can modify any of the melt and pour recipes to suit a hand-milled soap as well.

Simple Exfoliating Bar

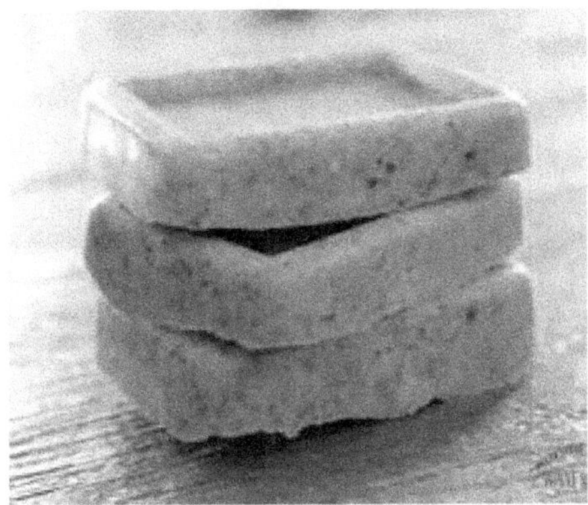

This bar is a perfect example of how you can take a clear melt and pour base and turn it into a customized spa bar. The exfoliants gently brush away dry skin, and the coffee invigorates and conditions. Yields up to four bars, depending on the size and shape of your molds.

Ingredients:

- 2 cups melt and pour soap base, grated
- ½ cup almonds, finely ground
- 2 teaspoons coffee grounds
- 15-20 drops sweet orange essential oil

Directions:

1. Follow the instructions provided for melt and pour soap.

Melt and Pour Tropical Oasis Bar

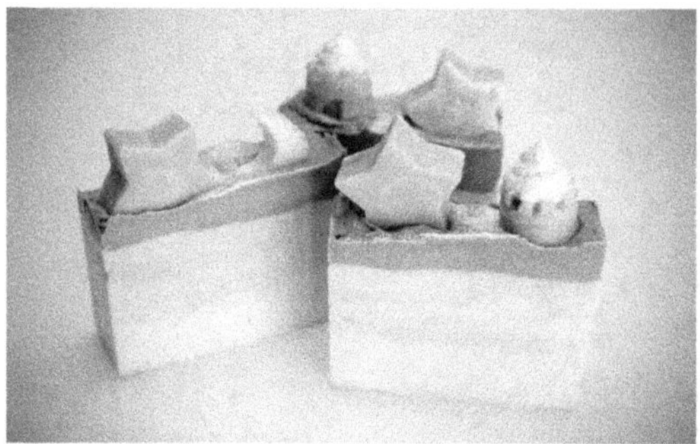

This bar will instantly take you away to the tropical oasis of your dreams. Laced with coconut, citrus, and jasmine, this makes for the perfect summertime bar. Yields up to four bars, depending upon the size and shape of your molds.

Ingredients:

- 2 cups melt and pour soap base, grated
- ¼ cup almonds, finely ground
- ¼ cup shredded coconut, finely grated
- 1 tablespoon lime zest
- 10 drops lime essential oil
- 5 drops jasmine essential oil

Directions:

1. Follow the instructions provided for melt and pour soap.

Garden Mint Bar

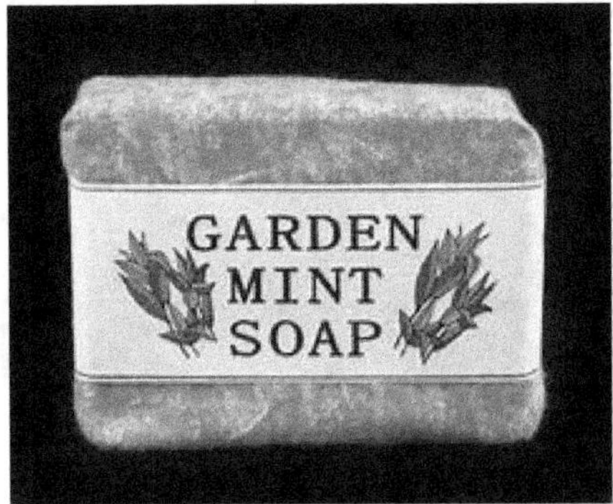

This refreshing mint bar is a perfect reminder of a fresh herb garden. This bar makes a good soap for both warm and cold weather, with the addition of soothing powdered milk. Yields up to four bars, depending upon the size and shape of your molds.

Ingredients:

- 2 cups melt and pour soap base
- ½ cup powdered milk
- ½ cup dried mint leaves, finely ground
- 10 drops peppermint essential oil
- 5 drops rosemary essential oil

Directions:

1. Follow the instructions provided for melt and pour soap.

Chocolate-Covered Fruit Bar

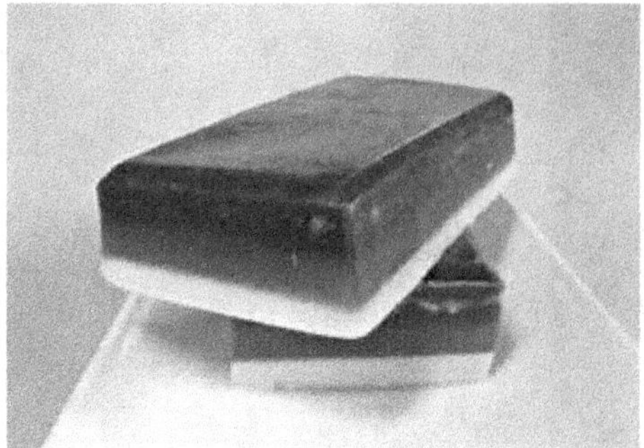

This bar is truly decadent and so mouth-watering that you will need to include instructions not to eat it! Yields up to four bars depending upon the size and shape of your molds.

Ingredients:

- 2 cups melt and pour soap base, grated
- ¼ cup powdered milk
- 1 teaspoon cocoa powder
- 1 tablespoon candied orange peel, chopped.
- 10 drops sweet orange essential oil
- 5 drops peppermint essential oil

Directions:

1. Follow the instructions provided for melt and pour soap.

Spicy Shower Bar

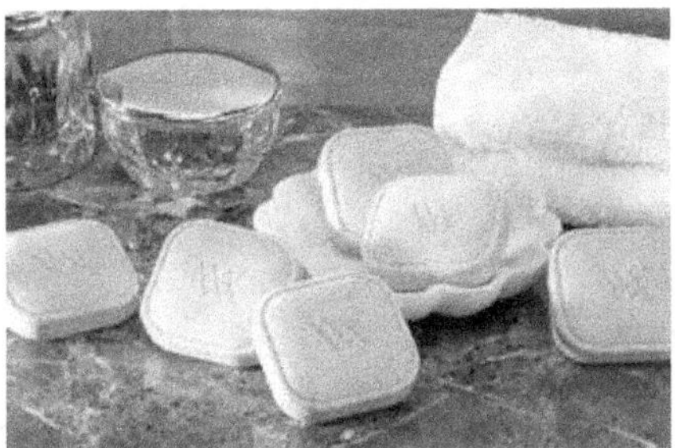

This bar makes a wonderful gift for the men in your life or anyone who prefers a more earthy and spicy smelling soap. The honey and powdered milk are moisturizing, while the herbs are healing and soothing. Yields approximately four bars depending on the size and shape of your molds.

Ingredients:

- 2 cups melt and pour soap base, grated
- ¼ cup powdered milk
- 2 teaspoons honey
- 1 teaspoon ground sage
- 1 teaspoon dried basil
- 2 teaspoons fresh rosemary, ground
- 5 drops cinnamon essential oil
- 10 drops rosemary essential oil

Directions:

1. Follow the instructions provided for melt and pour soap.

Sweet Honey Bar

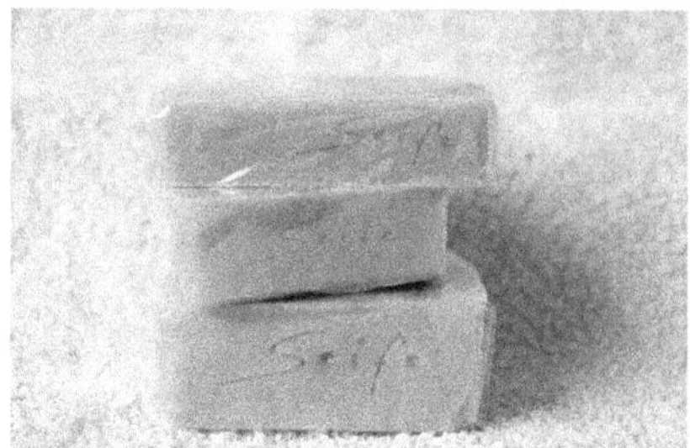

You can add nourishing ingredients such as honey, wheat germ, and oatmeal to your melt and pour soap base to create the soap that looks, feels, and smells like a unique bar. Yields approximately four bars of soap depending on the size and shape of your mold.

Ingredients:

- 2 cups melt and pour soap base
- 2 tablespoons beeswax pellets
- 2 tablespoons honey
- 1 tablespoon wheat germ
- 1 tablespoon oatmeal, finely ground
- 10 drops bergamot essential oil

Directions:

1. Follow the instructions provided for melt and pour soap.

Chapter 4 – Other Soaps

Peppermint and Tea Tree Oil Acne Soap

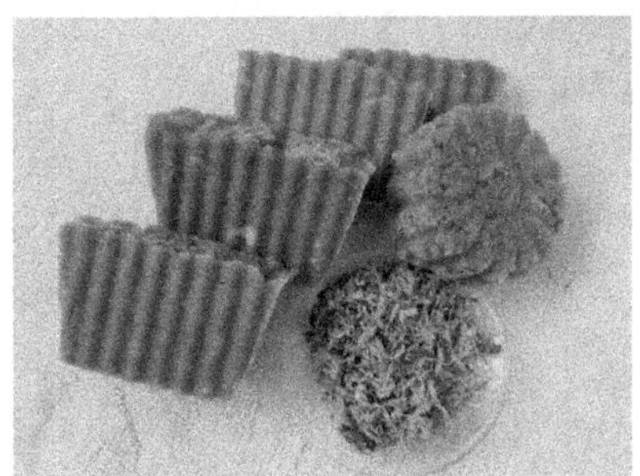

Most over-the-counter acne medicines, cleansers, and soaps are full of strong chemicals. Unfortunately, many people mistake this as being a good thing. They think that they need harsh chemicals to kill their blemishes and that the key to curing acne is to dry out their skin.

This couldn't be further from the truth. In reality, drying your skin makes it produce even more oil, which in turn produces more pimples. Strong chemicals inflame the skin and make it dry and flaky. This acne soap is gentle yet contains natural ingredients that prevent breakouts. Coconut oil is an antibacterial that kills the bacteria in/on your skin that causes acne. Neem oil is also an anti-bacterial and helps reduce redness and inflammation caused by acne. Tea tree oil works as well as prescription drugs like benzoyl peroxide to remedy pimples. Castor oil cleans pores by pulling out excess oils and bacteria. Olive oil is an antioxidant, which helps reduce the appearance of acne scars.

This soap is safe and ready for use after it hardens.

Ingredients:

- Peppermint Essential Oil (1 oz.)
- Tea Tree Oil (1 oz.)
- Lye (4 ½ oz.)
- Water (10 oz.)
- Organic Cold-pressed Olive Oil (10 oz.)
- Organic, Unrefined, Cold-pressed Coconut Oil (10 oz.)
- Organic Castor Oil (2 oz.)
- Organic Palm Oil (3 oz.)
- Organic Neem Oil (6 oz.)
- Beeswax (2 oz.)

Directions:

1. Pour water into a large stainless steel or glass bowl.
2. Pour lye into water, stirring it until the lye has dissolved.
3. Fill a large bowl halfway with cold water and ice cubes. Place the bowl with water and lye into this larger bowl. Make sure that the water and lye mixture stays cold. If the ice melts, add more.
4. Pour beeswax and olive oil, coconut oil, castor oil, palm oil, and neem oil into a pot. Heat them on medium-low heat on the stove until they've all melted.
5. Transfer the beeswax and oil mixture into a crockpot. Heat on the lowest setting.
6. Slowly pour the lye and water into the crockpot. Stir until well mixed.
7. Use the stick blender to blend the mixture in the crockpot. Blend for three to five minutes. By then it should reach trace.

8.   Place the lid on the crockpot and leave the mixture covered for at least one hour while on lowest heat setting. The mixture should look a bit translucent.

9.   Add peppermint oil and tea tree oil to the mixture.

10.   Pour mixture into soap molds.

11.   After 24 hours, remove from the molds and cut it into bars. If they're still not completely hard, leave them uncovered for a few hours.

Neem Oil Soap for Psoriasis

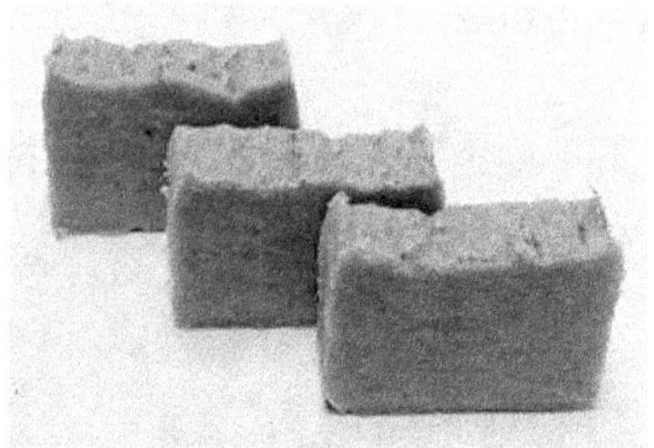

Psoriasis flare-ups can be very painful. Many people feel embarrassed of the dry red patches that populate their skin during a psoriasis outbreak. Neem oil has been used to clear up the patches brought up by psoriasis. Because it's an emollient, neem oil can soften the scaly, dry patches of skin caused by a psoriasis flare-up. It also soothes the itchiness and can reduce redness. Try this soap if you have psoriasis and are in need of soothing an outbreak.

Ingredients:

- Organic Neem Oil (3 ½ oz.)
- Lye (4 $\frac{9}{10}$ oz.)
- Distilled Water (12 oz.)
- Organic Argan Oil (1 $\frac{3}{10}$ oz.)
- Organic, Unrefined, Cold-pressed Coconut Oil (3⅗ oz.)
- OrganicCold-pressed Olive Oil (4⅗ oz.)
- Organic Apricot Kernel Oil (3⅗ oz.)
- Organic Tamanu Oil (1 oz.)
- Organic Wheat Germ Oil (1 $\frac{3}{10}$ oz.)

- Organic Cocoa Butter (1 $\frac{3}{10}$ oz.)
- Organic Grape Seed Oil (10⅘ oz.)
- Organic Shea Butter (1 $\frac{3}{10}$ oz.)
- Organic Palm Kernel Flakes (7⅕ oz.)

Directions:

1. Pour water into a large stainless steel or glass bowl.
2. Pour lye into water, stirring it until the lye has dissolved.
3. Fill a large bowl halfway with cold water and ice cubes. Place the bowl with water and lye into this larger bowl. Make sure that the water and lye mixture stays cold. If the ice melts, add more.
4. Pour the cocoa butter, shea butter, and the argan oil, coconut oil, olive oil, apricot kernel oil, tamanu oil, wheat germ oil, and palm kernel flakes into the non-aluminum pot. Heat them on the stove on medium heat. Once everything has melted, take the pot off of the stove. Set it aside and leave it to cool down.
5. Allow the butter and oil mixture and the water and lye mixture to cool down until they're between 110 and 115 degrees Fahrenheit.
6. Pour the water and lye into the butter and oil mixture. Blend with a stick blender until it begins to thicken and reaches trace.
7. Pour the neem oil into the mixture. Stir it in until it's well blended.
8. Pour the mixture into soap mold. Cover the mold and let it sit for at least 24 hours.
9. Remove soap from the mold and cut it into bars. Let the bars cure for a minimum of three weeks.

Winter Foot Soap Soak

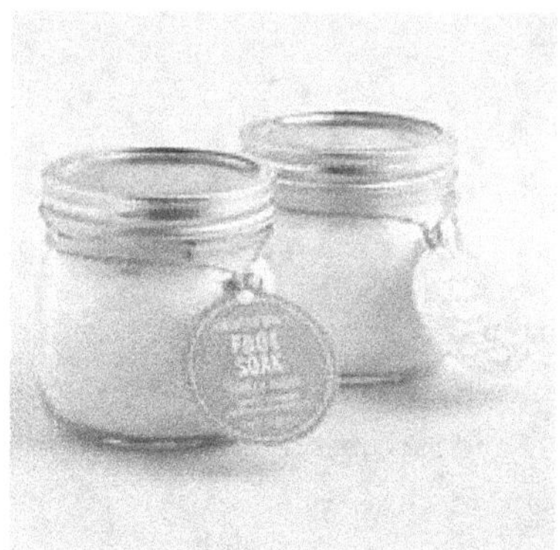

When your feet are feeling frigid due to plummeting winter temperatures, this sudsy DIY foot soak is sure to warm them up.

Ingredients:

- ¼ c. lemon juice
- ¼ c. milk
- 3 tbsps. extra virgin olive oil
- 1 tbsp. castile soap
- 1/8 tsp. cinnamon

Directions:

Place all ingredients in a large basin and add hot warm. Give the solution a stir with your hand, and allow your feet to soak for as long as you like.

Happy Winter Skin Facial Soap

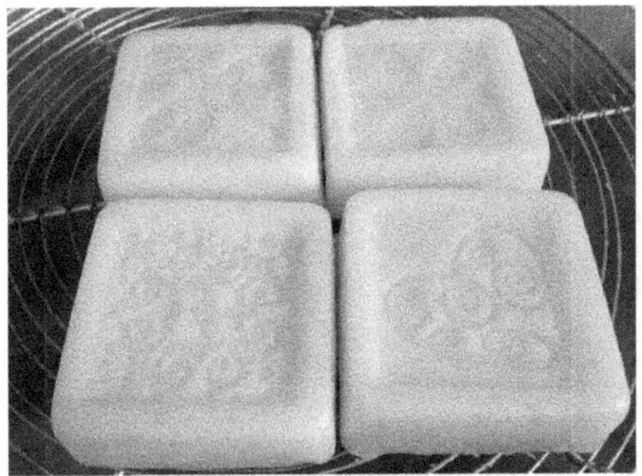

Is your face dried out due to frosty winter air? Treat yourself to this moisture-rich facial soap.

Ingredients:

- 2 apple slices, peeled
- ½ c. plain yogurt
- ½ c. tbsp. olive oil
- ½ tbsp. raw honey

Directions:

Blend all ingredients in a food processor or blender until smooth and creamy. Massage soap onto skin and allow to sit for 5-minutes. Rinse with warm water.

Moisturizing Honey Shower Wash

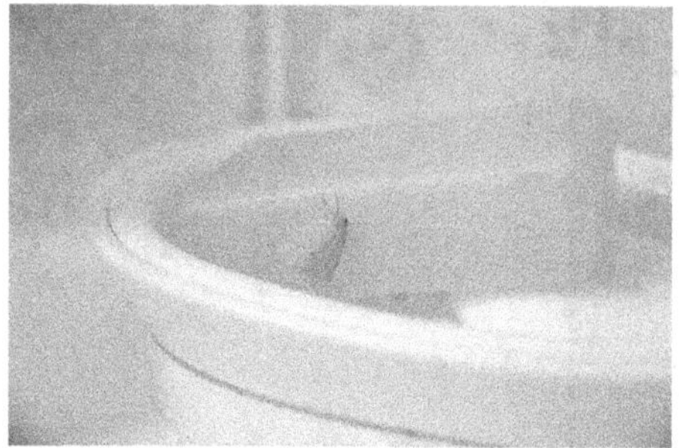

Ingredients:

- 2/3 c. castile soap
- ¼ c. raw honey
- 2 tbsp. grapeseed oil
- 1 tsp. vitamin E oil
- 50 – 60 drops vanilla essential oil

Directions:

Place all ingredients in a recycled shampoo or body wash container and shake vigorously. Squirt onto a washcloth or loofah.

Homemade Dish Soap

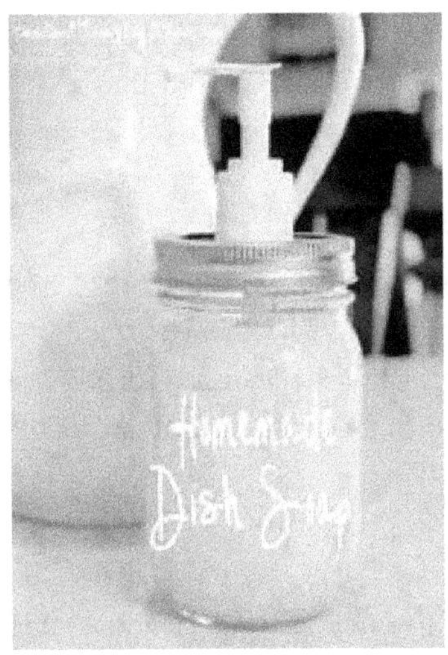

Ingredients:

- 1 ¾ c. boiling water
- 1 tbsp. borax
- 1 tbsp. grated Ivory or Castile bar soap
- 15 – 20 drops of orange or lemon essential oil

Directions:

Heat water until boiling. Next, add the borax and grated bar soap to a medium bowl. Then, pour the boiled water over the top of the soap mixture. Whisk until the soap dissolves. Allow the mixture to cool for about 8 hours, stirring now and then. Transfer the dish soap to a squirt bottle and add in the essential oil. Shake well to combine.

Conclusion

Washing your body shouldn't be treated as a chore. Instead, it should be treated as a ritual. You should find enjoyment, satisfaction, and pleasure in bathing. Take the time to really feel the textures of these unique soaps on your skin. Slow down and deeply inhale their aromas.

Your body is special and important. Washing with homemade organic soap is so much better for your skin, mind and spirit than using a commercial soap! You deserve so much more than artificial fragrances and toxic chemicals. You deserve nourishing ingredients that soothe the skin, delight the senses, and stimulate the mind.

Now that you see the positive effect that natural soaps can have on your skin, you should continue your soap education. Research new fragrances and additives that you can put in your soap. Think hard about what feelings you want to evoke when you shower. Think hard about what your skin needs. Does it need more moisture? Do you have a rash? Learn about more ingredients that can repair your skin.

Continue to think about the ingredients in your soap, and also in the environment around you. Read labels, ask questions. Is this good for me? Is there a harmful ingredient in this?

Now that you know that soap making is a fun, fulfilling activity, we hope that you continue to make soaps for yourselves and for the people you love. Share your creations with others. Tell them to take a long shower with one of your soaps and ask them if they notice a difference in their skin, body, mind, and spirit.